THE HORMONE FIX

BOOK

Hormonal Balance Support for Enhanced Well-being

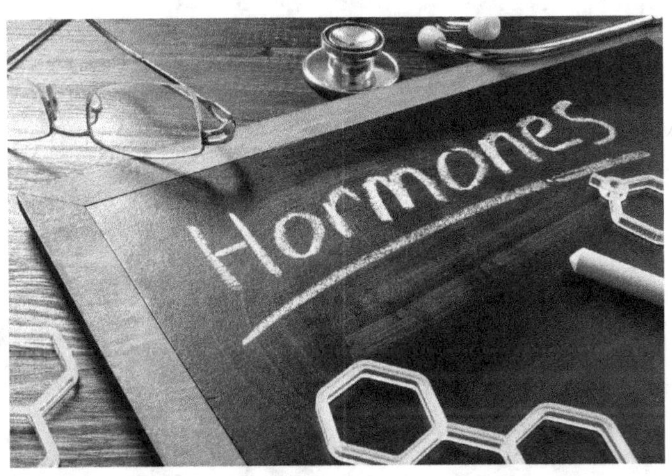

Mildred R. Thomas

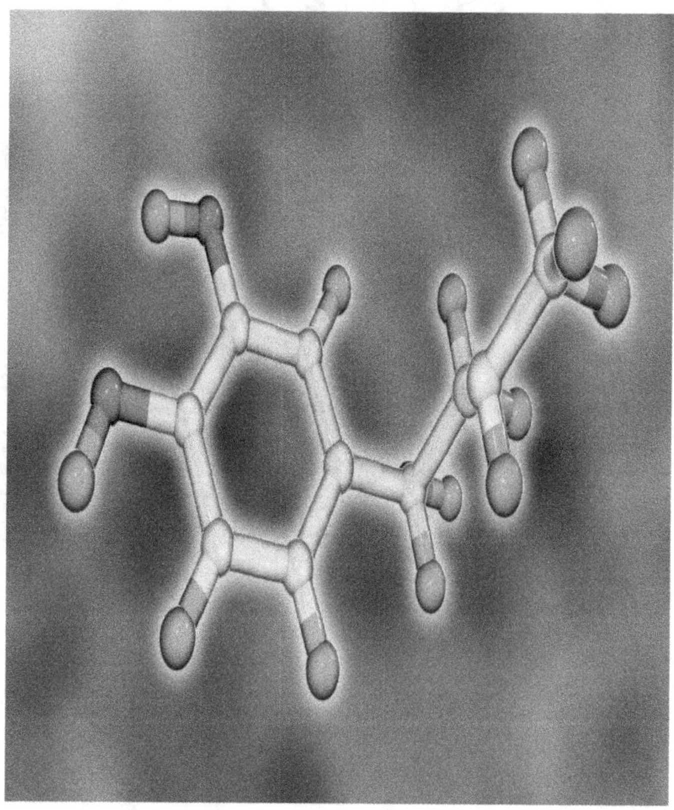

TABLE OF CONTENTS

Introduction

Senam, a vivacious young woman in her mid-twenties, resided in the small hamlet of Crestwood, tucked amid rolling hills and a babbling brook. Senam had always been full of life, with contagious laughter and limitless energy. However, in recent months, she had developed an unexplainable lethargy, casting a shadow over her previously exuberant existence. Fatigue seized her like a phantom, and a mist of malaise obscured her daily activities. Senam sought answers from numerous medical authorities, but the elusive source of her illness remained a mystery.

Senam discovered a ray of hope in an unlikely location one dismal afternoon, as rains tapped lightly against her bedroom window—a dusty old bookstore on the outskirts of town. She pushed open the creaking door with purpose, and the chiming of a little bell signaled her arrival. The small shop, with its weathered wooden shelves and the smell of old paper, appeared to be locked in time. Senam was walking through the short aisles when she discovered a strange book that drew her in with an almost magnetic force.

The title was embossed in gold letters and stated "Fix Your Hormones: A Comprehensive Guide to Restoring Balance." Senam, intrigued, picked up the book and began flipping through its pages. Each chapter offered insights into the complicated dance of hormones within the body, as well as solutions to a slew of health conditions that she was experiencing. It was as if the universe had brought her here, offering her a lifeline in the form of knowledge.

Dr. Amelia Hartwell was a well-known endocrinologist whose knowledge of hormonal health has changed the lives of countless people. Senam uncovered a universe of interrelated systems and delicate balances that influenced everything from mood to metabolism as she went into the pages. Dr. Hartwell's writing was straightforward and caring, and it spoke directly to Senam's heart, as if the doctor herself knew her difficulties.

Senam chose to go on a road of self-discovery and healing with renewed zeal. She began implementing the prescribed lifestyle modifications and food adjustments mentioned in the "Fix Your Hormones" book as her guide. The importance of full, nutrient-dense diets, frequent exercise, and stress management as cornerstones of hormonal well-being was underlined in the book. Senam embraced these concepts wholeheartedly, aiming to recapture the vibrancy that had been missing from her for far too long.

Senam's metamorphosis became obvious as the weeks passed. The cloud of fatigue gradually dissipated, showing the muted glitter in her eyes. She incorporated healthful meals into her regular regimen, appreciating the rich colors and textures prescribed by Dr. Hartwell. Senam developed a fresh love for yoga, finding consolation in its gentle motions and the mental peace it provided. Her constant companion was the book, its pages dog-eared and scribbled with her comments and development.

Senam's journey was not without difficulties. There were times when she felt frustrated and unsure, but the knowledge she received from "Fix Your Hormones" became her rock. Dr. Hartwell's remarks served as a guiding light, reminding Senam that recovery was a lengthy process, and every single step mattered. She found encouragement and understanding in internet networks where others had gone through similar experiences.

Senam's laughter and enthusiasm for life returned as her vitality restored. Crestwood residents couldn't help but notice their once-weary neighbor's miraculous transformation. Senam became a source of encouragement for others who, like her, had faced the formidable problem of hormone imbalance.

The dusty old bookstore in the heart of Crestwood witnessed a magnificent story of resilience and restoration. Senam's journey, propelled by the knowledge gained in "Fix Your Hormones," became a testament to the power of knowledge and the tremendous impact it can have on one's well-being. The book, long lost on a shelf, had become a catalyst for Senam's transformation—a triumphant story that rang through Crestwood's hills and valleys, motivating others to start on their own paths of healing and self-discovery.

CHAPTER 1: THE HORMONE FIX REVOLUTION

The Importance of Hormones

Hormones have a vital role in many biological processes, such as growth and development, metabolism, immunological response, mood regulation, and reproduction.

Control of Metabolism: The pancreas secretes hormones including insulin, which are essential for controlling blood glucose levels. Insulin helps cells absorb glucose, which contributes to steady blood sugar levels. Thyroid hormones control how much energy the body uses, which has an impact on metabolism.

Growth and Development: Normal growth and development depend on growth hormones, such as human growth hormone (HGH). They ensure that youngsters grow into healthy adults by promoting the growth of bones and tissues. These hormones still contribute to the maintenance of bone and muscle mass in adults.

Reproductive Functions: The development of secondary sexual traits and the control of the menstrual cycle depend on sex hormones, specifically testosterone in men and estrogen and progesterone in women. These hormones are also essential for the growth of reproductive organs and fertility.

Stress Reaction: In reaction to stress, hormones such as cortisol are released. Because they raise blood sugar, depress the immune system, and facilitate the metabolism of lipids, proteins, and carbs, they contribute to the body's "fight or flight" response.

Immune System Regulation: The growth and function of the immune system are influenced by certain hormones, including thymosin. Despite being well-known for its impact on stress, cortisol also suppresses the immune system.

Mood Regulation: Hormones have an impact on emotional health and mood. Serotonin, for instance—often referred to as the "feel-good" hormone—affects disorders like anxiety and depression and is involved in mood regulation.

Fluid and Electrolyte Balance: The body's fluid and electrolyte balance is regulated by hormones such as antidiuretic hormone (ADH) and aldosterone. They affect the kidneys' ability to reabsorb water and electrolytes, which helps to maintain enough hydration.

Maintenance of Homeostasis: Hormones have a role in maintaining homeostasis, which is the general equilibrium and stability of the body's internal environment. In order to guarantee ideal physiological function, they aid in controlling blood pressure, temperature, and other essential factors.

The Signs of Hormonal Imbalance

Recognizing Symptoms

1. Fatigue and Low Energy: Excessive weariness and a lack of energy may indicate hormone abnormalities.
2. Mood Swings:Mood swings or rapid shifts in emotions may be caused by hormone variations.
3. Irregular Menstrual Cycles: Hormonal disruptions can occur in women who have irregular periods or changes in menstrual cycles.
4. Difficulty or Weight Gain Losing Weight: Hormonal imbalances can interfere with metabolism, resulting in weight problems.
5. Insomnia or Poor Sleep Quality: Because hormones play a role in sleep regulation, disturbances may result in insomnia or restless nights.
6. Night sweats and hot flashes are common signs of hormonal abnormalities, particularly in menopausal women.

7. Reduced Libido: Hormonal imbalances can have an effect on sexual desire and function.

8. Hair Loss or Thinning: Hormone fluctuations can cause hair loss or thinning in both men and women.

9. Difficulty concentrating, memory lapses, and mental fogginess are all symptoms of hormone swings.

10. Hormonal imbalances can influence digestion, causing symptoms such as bloating, gas, or constipation.

11. Skin Changes: Acne, dry skin, and other skin disorders may be signs of hormonal imbalances.

12. Inflammation and joint discomfort can be exacerbated by hormonal abnormalities.

13. Stress Sensitivity:Hormones regulate the body's stress response, and abnormalities can lead to increased stress sensitivity.

14. PMS (Premenstrual Syndrome) Symptoms:Due to hormonal fluctuations, women may have heightened premenstrual symptoms.

15. Muscle Mass Loss:Hormonal changes, particularly in the elderly, can contribute to a loss of muscle mass and strength.

Physical Signs

1. Changes of the Skin: Acne, dryness, or increased sensitivity of the skin.
2. Thinning or excessive shedding of hair.
3. Weight gain: Particularly around the midsection.
4. Fatigue is defined as persistent exhaustion and a lack of energy.
5. Mood swings are unexplained emotional swings.
6. Hot flashes are short bursts of intense heat.
7. Excessive sweating while sleeping is referred to as night sweats.
8. Menstrual Cycle Irregularities: Changes in timing, flow, or duration.
9. Insomnia is defined as difficulty falling or staying asleep.
10. Difficulty concentrating or memory lapses are symptoms of brain fog.
11. Libido changes: decreased interest in sex.
12. Breast Tenderness: Pain or swelling in the breasts.
13. Bloating, constipation, or diarrhea are all symptoms of digestive problems.

14. Joint pain refers to aches and discomfort in the joints.

15. Headaches: Severe or frequent headaches.

16. Appetite Changes: Increased or decreased hunger.

17. Allergies: Increased sensitivity to allergens.

18. Muscle Weakness: The sensation of being physically weaker than usual.

19. Increased Thirst: Feelings of dehydration that persist.

20. Elevated Heart Rate: Changes in heart rate or palpitations that are noticeable.

Emotional and Mental Signs

1. Mood Swings: Hormonal variations can cause abrupt and strong mood swings, making emotional regulation difficult.

2. Anxiety and Restlessness: Cortisol and adrenaline imbalances may contribute to anxiety and a prolonged sense of restlessness.

3. Depression and poor Mood: Hormone and serotonin fluctuations can lead to emotions of melancholy, despair, and chronic poor mood.

4. Irritation and fury: Hormone imbalances, particularly during PMS or menopause, can cause irritation and unexpected spurts of fury.

5. Forgetfulness and Brain Fog: Hormonal imbalances can impair cognitive function, resulting in difficulty with attention, memory lapses, and general brain fog.

6. Insomnia and Sleep Disturbances: Melatonin and progesterone level disruptions may lead to problems falling or staying asleep, affecting general mental well-being.

7. Fatigue and Low Energy: Hormonal abnormalities, such as thyroid dysfunction, can cause persistent fatigue and low energy levels, which can have an impact on motivation and mood.

8. Libido fluctuations: Changes in testosterone and estrogen levels can alter sexual desire, resulting in libido and overall pleasure fluctuations.

9. Panic Attacks: Hormonal imbalances, notably cortisol and adrenaline, can contribute to panic attacks or heightened stress responses.

10. Increased Stress Sensitivity: Hormones play an important part in the body's stress response, and

abnormalities can result in increased sensitivity to stressors.

11. Emotional Eating: Hormonal variations, particularly in insulin and cortisol, might lead to emotional eating behaviors as a stress and mood swing coping technique.

12. Hormonal imbalances can cause feelings of loneliness and a tendency to retreat from social engagements.

13. Loss of Motivation: Dopamine and serotonin imbalances can affect the brain's reward system, resulting in a loss of motivation and interest in activities.

14. Emotional Sensitivity Increased: Hormonal changes can increase emotional reactions, making people more emotionally sensitive to diverse stimuli.

15. Difficulty Coping with Change: Hormonal imbalances can make it difficult to cope with life changes or unexpected events.

16. Hormone imbalances can lead to poor stress coping techniques, such as increased alcohol or drug usage.

17. Excessive Worrying: Hormonal abnormalities, particularly cortisol imbalances, may contribute to persistent worrying and elevated anxiety levels.

18. Lack of Emotional Resilience: Hormonal balance is important for emotional resilience, and abnormalities can lead to a diminished capacity to recover from life's hardships.

19. Inability to Focus: Hormone fluctuations can disrupt neurotransmitters, affecting focus and attention span.

20. Overload: Hormonal imbalances can lead to feelings of overload, making it difficult to negotiate everyday chores and obligations.

Hormones in Adolescence

1. The Hormonal Symphony: Adolescence is a time of increased hormonal activity, during which the endocrine system orchestrates a symphony of changes. A rise in hormones, principally estrogen and testosterone, causes puberty, the doorway to adolescent. These chemical messengers play a critical role in developing physical traits ranging from growth

spurts and the development of secondary sexual characteristics to reproductive organ maturation.

2. Emotional Rollercoaster:Hormone surges affect more than just the body; they also have a significant impact on emotions and behavior. Adolescents are frequently on an emotional rollercoaster, with mood swings, increased sensitivity, and powerful emotional responses. The delicate interplay of hormones such as cortisol, adrenaline, and serotonin is responsible for this rollercoaster ride.

3. Hormones also play an important influence in the development of the teenage brain. During this time, the prefrontal cortex, which is responsible for decision-making and impulse control, develops significantly. Hormones like insulin-like growth factor (IGF) and brain-derived neurotrophic factor (BDNF) help to shape the brain's structure, influencing cognitive capacities and emotional regulation.

4. Hormones and Identity Formation: Hormones play a role in the development of identity and personality as teenagers walk the route to self-discovery. The increase in sex hormones not

only causes bodily changes, but it also has an impact on sexual orientation, gender identity, and the establishment of romantic relationships. This stage is distinguished by a desire for autonomy and a better knowledge of one's role in the world.

5. Adolescent hormone fluctuations are a natural component of growth, but they can provide difficulties for both teenagers and their caretakers. Family conflicts can be exacerbated by mood swings, impatience, and risk-taking behavior. Understanding the molecular roots of these behaviors, on the other hand, can develop empathy and open communication.

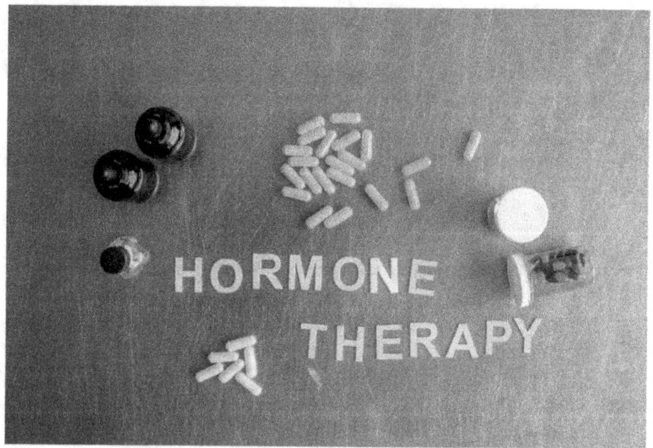

The Benefits of Hormone Optimization

Enhanced Vitality:
Energy metabolism is influenced by hormones, including thyroid and cortisol. Enhancing these hormones can result in more vitality overall, less weariness, and more energy.

Improved Emotion and Mental Health:
Stress and mood are largely controlled by hormones including cortisol, dopamine, and serotonin. Stabilizing and improving mental health may be aided by hormone balance.

Improved Quality of Sleep:
Hormones that control the sleep-wake cycle include cortisol and melatonin. Hormone optimization can

enhance the quality of sleep, resulting in more revitalizing and peaceful slumber.

Strength and Muscle Mass:

Growth hormone and testosterone are necessary for the growth and maintenance of muscle. Strengthening and lean muscle mass growth can be aided by optimizing these hormones.

Maintaining a Healthy Weight:

Insulin and leptin are two examples of hormones that influence hunger and metabolism. Reducing the risk of obesity and improving weight management can be achieved by balancing these hormones.

Ideal Health of Bones:

For the purpose of preserving bone density and averting diseases like osteoporosis, hormones like estrogen, testosterone, and vitamin D are essential. Optimizing hormones can promote bone health and lower the chance of fractures.

Enhanced Sexual and Libido Function:

In both men and women, libido and sexual function are strongly correlated with hormones such as testosterone. Enhancing sexual performance and desire might result from hormone balance.

Mental Process:

Estrogen and testosterone, for example, are linked to cognitive function and have neuroprotective properties. Improving hormone levels may help with focus, memory, and general cognitive wellness.

Heart Health:

Blood artery function, cholesterol levels, and blood pressure are all influenced by hormones. Optimizing hormone levels can help maintain cardiovascular health and lower the chance of developing heart-related problems.

Improved Skin Conditions:

Hormones affect the elasticity, formation of collagen, and secretion of oil from the skin. Enhancing hormone levels can help promote younger-looking, healthier skin.

Enhanced Immune Response:

Immune response modulation is influenced by hormones. Hormone balance can support a healthy immune system and lessen vulnerability to infections and diseases.

Lower Chance of Chronic Illnesses:
A lower chance of developing several chronic illnesses, such as diabetes, osteoporosis, and cardiovascular diseases, has been associated with hormone optimization.

Relieving Menopausal Symptoms:
By raising estrogen and progesterone levels, hormone optimization, especially through hormone replacement therapy (HRT), can reduce menopausal symptoms such hot flashes, night sweats, and mood swings.

Improved Outcomes during Exercise:
Hormone optimization, such as testosterone optimization, can lead to improved muscular endurance and recovery, which in turn can improve exercise performance and capacity.

Decreased Inflammation:

The body's inflammatory response can be influenced by hormones. Hormone balance has the potential to reduce chronic inflammation, which has been connected to a number of illnesses, such as arthritis and cardiovascular disease.

Enhanced Metabolic Function:
By improving insulin sensitivity and glucose metabolism, hormone optimization can lower the risk of insulin resistance and type 2 diabetes.

Menstrual cycles that are regulated:
For women to have regular menstrual periods, hormonal balance is essential. Polycystic ovarian syndrome and irregular periods can both be treated with hormone optimization, which also helps to regulate the menstrual cycle (PCOS).

Reduction of Symptoms of Andropause:
Aging men may see a drop in testosterone levels, similar to menopause, which can cause symptoms including exhaustion, decreased libido, and mood swings. Hormone optimization is a treatment option for these

symptoms in a disease known as male menopause or andropause.

Preventing Joint and Muscle Pain:

Muscle and joint health are influenced by hormones. Hormone optimization can lower the chance of aging-related muscle and joint discomfort as well as help prevent or treat diseases like arthritis.

Assistance with Thyroid Function:

The hormones that control metabolism are produced by the thyroid gland. Thyroid abnormalities can be addressed with hormone optimization, which will increase energy and metabolism.

Enhanced Recovery from Injuries:

Growth hormone in particular is involved in tissue repair and wound healing. Improving hormone levels can hasten the healing process following operations or accidents.

Guarding Against Mental Decline:

Estrogen is one hormone that has neuroprotective properties that may help prevent cognitive decline and diseases like Alzheimer's. Hormone optimization might help people maintain their cognitive abilities as they age.

Better Health of the Hair and Nails:
Hormones affect the growth of nails and hair. Hormone balance can help promote healthier hair and nails by lowering problems like brittle nails and hair loss.

Improved Standard of Living:
All things considered, the combined benefits of hormone optimization raise one's standard of living. When hormone levels are within optimal ranges, people frequently report feeling more alert, balanced, and energized.

The personalized medicine approach
Individual needs are frequently taken into consideration while optimizing hormones, and this includes things like age, gender, heredity, and general health. This tailored strategy may produce more focused and efficient outcomes.

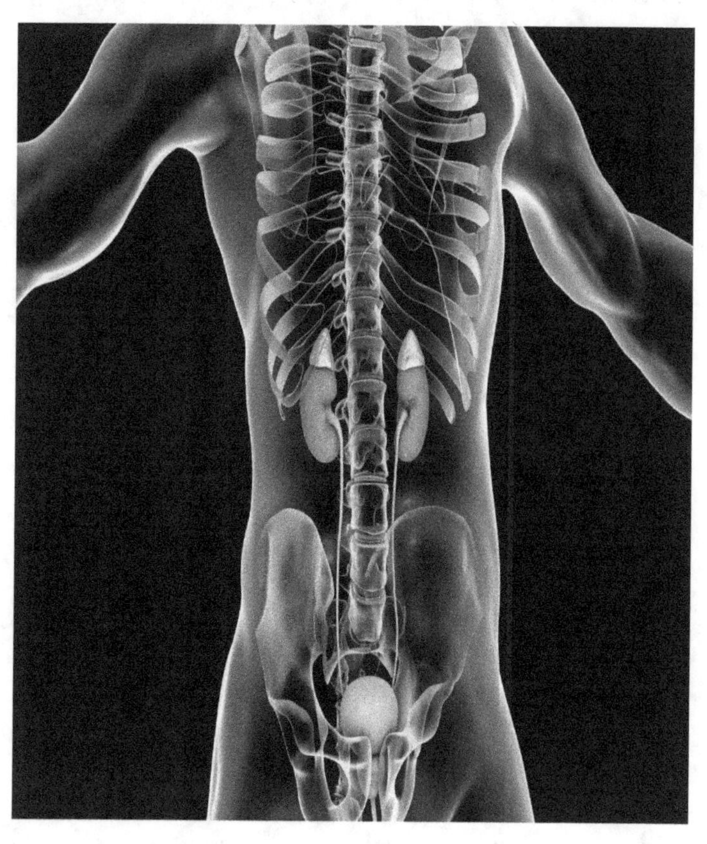

CHAPTER 2: THE MAJOR HORMONES AND THEIR FUNCTIONS

The Master Gland: The Pituitary Gland

The pituitary gland, sometimes known as the "master gland," is a pea-sized organ at the base of the brain. Despite its small size, this gland is critical in controlling many physiological systems throughout the body. It is frequently regarded as the endocrine system's commander-in-chief, directing the release of hormones that govern many other glands and organs.

The pituitary gland is separated into two parts: anterior pituitary (in front) and posterior pituitary (in back). Each portion is in charge of releasing certain hormones, which influence various elements of biological activities.

Pituitary Gland:
Growth hormone (GH), thyroid-stimulating hormone (TSH), adrenocorticotropic hormone (ACTH), follicle-stimulating hormone (FSH), luteinizing hormone (LH), and prolactin are all produced and released by the anterior pituitary gland.

Growth Hormone (GH): Promotes bone and tissue growth and development.

Thyroid-Stimulating Hormone (TSH): Controls thyroid gland activity, altering metabolism and energy levels.
ADH stimulates the adrenal glands to create cortisol, which is vital for stress response and metabolism.

Follicle-Stimulating Hormone (FSH) and Luteinizing Hormone (LH): These hormones influence the ovaries and testes and play important roles in the reproductive system.

Prolactin is a hormone that stimulates milk production in the mammary glands.

Posterior Pituitary Gland:

The posterior pituitary gland stores and releases hypothalamic hormones such as oxytocin and vasopressin (antidiuretic hormone).

Oxytocin is a hormone that increases milk ejection during breastfeeding and plays an important role in uterine contractions during birthing. It also serves social and bonding purposes.

Vasopressin (Antidiuretic Hormone): This hormone regulates water balance by modulating water reabsorption in the kidneys.

The Thyroid Gland: The Energy Regulator

The thyroid gland, a small butterfly-shaped organ found near the base of the neck, regulates the body's energy metabolism. This endocrine gland generates hormones that affect a variety of physiological processes, including growth, development, and nutrition metabolism. Thyroxine (T4) and triiodothyronine (T3) are the two principal hormones secreted by the thyroid gland and are referred to collectively as thyroid hormones.

- Thyroid hormones play an important role in maintaining the body's energy balance. They have an impact on practically every cell in the body, controlling how quickly cells use oxygen and nutrients to make energy. Thyroid hormones accomplish this by modifying the basal metabolic rate (BMR), which is the amount of energy required by the body at rest to maintain basic physiological activities.

- One of the thyroid gland's main duties is to respond to signals from the pituitary gland, which releases thyroid-stimulating hormone (TSH). When the body requires more thyroid hormones, the pituitary gland releases TSH, which causes the thyroid gland to boost T3 and T4 production and release. This complicated feedback loop keeps the body's metabolic rate within an optimal range.

- Thyroid hormones regulate carbohydrate, lipid, and protein metabolism. They improve food absorption from the digestive tract, increase glycogen breakdown into glucose, and promote glucose use for energy production. Furthermore, these hormones play an important role in lipid metabolism, affecting fat breakdown and conversion into energy.

- Thyroid hormones are especially important during growth and development because they help tissues and organs mature. Adequate thyroid hormone levels in children are required for appropriate physical and mental development.

- When the thyroid gland malfunctions, either by producing too many (hyperthyroidism) or too few (hypothyroidism) thyroid hormones, energy control can be severely disrupted. Hyperthyroidism causes an elevated metabolic rate, which can cause symptoms such as weight loss, increased heart rate, and nervousness. Hypothyroidism, on the other hand, can cause a sluggish metabolism, resulting in symptoms such as weight gain, weariness, and cold intolerance.

- Thyroid function can be affected by a variety of factors, including dietary status, environmental impacts, and autoimmune illnesses. Iodine, an essential mineral, is required for the manufacture of thyroid hormones, and a lack of it can result in thyroid dysfunction.

The Adrenal Glands: The Stress Responders

The adrenal glands, which look like little triangular hats atop each kidney, play an important part in the body's response to stress. These extraordinary glands are critical components of the endocrine system, generating hormones that impact many physiological processes. One of its key jobs is to regulate the body's stress response by secreting chemicals such as cortisol and adrenaline. Understanding the complicated mechanics of the adrenal glands reveals how the body deals with stress and maintains balance.

- The Adrenal Glands: Anatomy
  The adrenal glands are divided into two parts: the outer adrenal cortex and the inner adrenal medulla. In response to diverse cues, each region releases different hormones. Corticosteroids, including cortisol, are synthesized in the adrenal cortex and are essential for regulating metabolism, immunological response, and blood pressure. The adrenal medulla, on the other hand, produces adrenaline (epinephrine) and

norepinephrine, which are hormones that swiftly prepare the body for the "fight or flight" reaction during stressful situations.

- When the body experiences stress, whether physical or psychological, the adrenal glands receive signals from the brain, specifically the hypothalamus and pituitary gland. This connection causes the adrenal cortex to release cortisol, also known as the "stress hormone." Cortisol mobilizes energy storage, raises blood sugar levels, and suppresses non-essential functions such as digestion, diverting resources to meet the stressor's immediate demands.

- Simultaneously, in response to stress signals, the adrenal medulla releases adrenaline and norepinephrine into the bloodstream. These hormones rapidly raise heart rate, dilate airways, and divert blood flow to vital organs and muscles, preparing the body to deal with or avoid the stressor. The adrenal glands' synchronized action ensures a quick and effective response to varied stressors, assisting the individual in adapting to difficult situations.

- Chronic Stress and Adrenal Fatigue: While the stress response is an important survival mechanism, prolonged exposure to stressors can result in chronic adrenal gland activation. This constant need for stress hormones may result in adrenal exhaustion or adrenal insufficiency. Adrena exhaustion can cause symptoms such as weariness, reduced immunological function, and trouble dealing with stress.

The Sex Hormones: Estrogen, Progesterone, and Testosterone

The sex hormones—estrogen, progesterone, and testosterone—play critical roles in the development and maintenance of both male and female sexual traits and reproductive activities. These hormones,are produced by the endocrine glands, predominantly the ovaries in females and the testes in males, though the adrenal glands also produce some.

Estrogen:

Estrogen is a female sex hormone that is responsible for the development and maintenance of female reproductive tissues as well as secondary sexual characteristics. It regulates the menstrual cycle, promotes the growth of the uterine lining, and influences bone density.

- Menstrual Cycle: During the menstrual cycle, estrogen levels rise, causing ovarian follicles to mature and the uterine lining to prepare for conception.

- Secondary Sexual Attributes: During puberty, estrogen leads to the growth of breast tissue, broader hips, and a more feminine body shape in general.

Progesterone:

Progesterone is another important female sex hormone that works in tandem with estrogen. It aids in the regulation of the menstrual cycle and is especially vital during pregnancy, where it aids in the formation of the placenta and the maintenance of the uterine lining.

- Menstrual Cycle: Progesterone levels rise after ovulation, preparing the uterine lining for a fertilized egg. If fertilization does not take place, progesterone levels fall, causing menstruation.
- Pregnancy: Progesterone is necessary for a healthy pregnancy because it prevents the uterus from contracting and promotes the growth of the placenta.

Testosterone:

While testosterone is commonly associated with males, it is present in both males and females, albeit in varying amounts. It is essential for the development of the male reproductive system, sperm production, and the development of male secondary sexual traits such as facial hair and a deeper voice in males.

Females generate testosterone in their ovaries and adrenal glands. It boosts libido, promotes bone health, and aids in the maintenance of general energy levels.

Puberty: During puberty, testosterone in males causes the Adam's apple to expand, muscle mass to develop, and face and body hair to sprout.

The Pancreas: The Insulin Producer

- The pancreas is a key organ in the human body that serves both digestive and endocrine functions. One of its most important tasks is the generation of insulin, a hormone necessary for blood sugar regulation. This little, elongated organ, snuggled beneath the stomach, is critical in maintaining glucose homeostasis, which ensures that the body's cells receive the energy they require to function properly.

- The pancreas is made up of two parts: the exocrine pancreas and the endocrine pancreas. The exocrine pancreas is in charge of manufacturing digestive enzymes that aid in food digestion in the small intestine. The endocrine pancreas, on the other hand, which accounts for only a small fraction of the organ, is engaged in the direct secretion of hormones into the bloodstream.

- The islets of Langerhans, which are clusters of cells within the endocrine pancreas, are where the magic of insulin manufacturing happens. These islets' principal cell types include alpha cells, beta cells, delta cells, and PP cells. The beta cell is of special significance when addressing insulin.

- In reaction to increased blood glucose levels, beta cells synthesize and secrete insulin. When a person consumes carbohydrates, the delicate dance of insulin release begins. As the digestive system converts these carbohydrates into glucose, this simple sugar enters the bloodstream.

- Beta cells release insulin into the bloodstream in response to rising blood glucose levels. Insulin functions like a key, unlocking cells and allowing glucose to enter. This promotes glucose uptake by various tissues, such as muscle and adipose (fat) tissue, where it is either used for energy or stored for later use. Concurrently, insulin restricts the liver's production and release of excess glucose into the bloodstream.

- Insulin's involvement in avoiding hyperglycemia, a disease defined by increased blood sugar levels, is critical. Chronic hyperglycemia can result in a number of health problems, including diabetes mellitus. Diabetes occurs when either the pancreas does not generate enough insulin (Type 1) or the body's cells become resistant to its effects (Type 2), resulting in poor glucose management.

- As a result, the pancreas acts as the body's watchful regulator, responding to the changing needs of glucose regulation. Its ability to manufacture and release insulin is critical to the delicate balance required for good cellular function and general health.

The Sleep Hormone: Melatonin

Melatonin, also known as the "sleep hormone," is a naturally occurring hormone in the human body that regulates sleep-wake cycles. Melatonin, which is produced by the pineal gland, a small pea-sized gland in the brain, is well-known for its important function in encouraging sleep and maintaining the body's circadian rhythm.

Sleep-Wake Cycle Regulation:
Melatonin secretion is strongly linked to the body's internal clock, or circadian rhythm. External elements such as light and darkness alter this rhythm. Melatonin production begins in the pineal gland in reaction to decreasing light levels, often in the evening as the day transitions into night. This increase in melatonin secretion tells the body that it is time to sleep.

External Factors:
Modern lifestyles, with greater exposure to artificial light, can interfere with melatonin production. Smartphones and computers, for example, emit blue light, which can suppress melatonin production and interfere with the body's ability to determine when it's

time to sleep. Creating a sleep-friendly environment in the evening by limiting exposure to bright lights and electronic devices can aid in the natural release of melatonin.

Supplementation and Health Advantages:
Melatonin pills are frequently used to treat sleep disorders like insomnia and jet lag. Melatonin supplements may also aid people who have inconsistent sleep habits or work night shifts. Melatonin may have antioxidant characteristics and may help the immune system, according to research, but more research is needed to fully grasp these potential health advantages.

CHAPTER 3: THE HORMONES IMBALANCES THAT CAN AFFECT YOU

Estrogen Dominance

Estrogen dominance is a condition in which the body's estrogen and progesterone levels are out of balance, with estrogen levels being disproportionately high in comparison to progesterone. Estrogen and progesterone are both hormones that play important functions in the menstrual cycle and overall hormonal homeostasis. Estrogen dominance can result from a variety of circumstances, including:

Excessive Estrogen Production: The body may create too much estrogen naturally or as a result of external causes such as exposure to estrogen-mimicking compounds in the environment (known as xenoestrogens), which can be found in some plastics and pollutants.

Inadequate Progesterone Production: A lack of progesterone, the hormone that balances estrogen's effects, can contribute to estrogen dominance. This can occur during specific phases of the menstrual cycle or as a result of disorders such as polycystic ovary syndrome (PCOS).

Impaired Estrogen Metabolism: Maintaining hormonal balance requires proper estrogen metabolism. If the body has trouble metabolizing estrogen, it can lead to estrogen buildup and contribute to estrogen dominance.

Estrogen dominance symptoms may include:
Menstrual periods that are irregular
Periods that are heavy or uncomfortable
Breast sensitivity
Swings in mood
Weight gain, particularly in the hips and thighs
Breast fibrocystic
Fatigue
Estrogen dominance can have a variety of health consequences for women, including an increased risk of endometriosis, fibroids, and some types of cancer.

Low Testosterone

Hypogonadism, or low testosterone, can cause hormonal abnormalities. Age, certain medical conditions, drugs, and lifestyle factors can all contribute to low testosterone levels. Here are a few examples of common causes:

- Testosterone levels naturally fall with age, usually beginning around middle life. This decline is a normal part of aging, but it can lead to symptoms including weariness, decreased libido, and mood changes.

- Medical problems: Certain medical problems can interfere with testosterone production. Obesity, diabetes, and hormonal imbalances can all contribute to low testosterone levels.

- Some medicines, such as corticosteroids and opiates, might inhibit testosterone synthesis.

- Testicular illnesses: Conditions that affect the testicles, such as injury, infection, or some genetic illnesses, can lead to insufficient testosterone.

- Long-term illnesses, particularly those affecting the endocrine system or pituitary gland, can disturb hormonal balance, including testosterone levels.

- Low testosterone can cause fatigue, decreased libido, erectile dysfunction, depression, and loss of muscular mass. It's crucial to remember that these symptoms might be caused by a variety of other conditions, so a healthcare professional should investigate and diagnose the underlying problem.

Treatment for low testosterone may include hormone replacement treatment (HRT) or treating underlying factors such as weight loss, chronic disease management, or prescription modifications. Changes in lifestyle, such as regular exercise, a good diet, and appropriate sleep, can help boost testosterone levels.

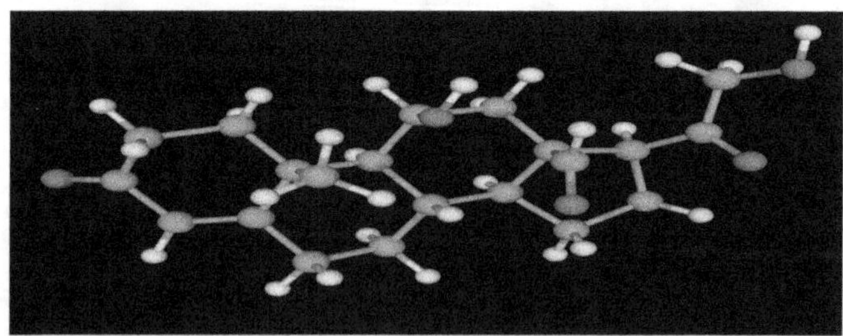

Thyroid Dysfunction

Thyroid dysfunction is a major contributor to hormonal imbalances in the body. The thyroid gland, which is located in the neck, generates hormones called triiodothyronine (T3) and thyroxine (T4), which regulate metabolism and influence a variety of physiological processes. When the thyroid gland fails to operate effectively, an imbalance in these hormones occurs, leading in a variety of health problems.

Hypothyroidism:
Hypothyroidism occurs when the thyroid gland does not generate adequate thyroid hormones. This can cause weariness, weight gain, cold sensitivity, and a sluggish metabolism.

Influence on Other Hormones: Thyroid hormone deficiency can throw off the balance of other hormones in the body. For example, it may result in increased levels of prolactin, a hormone involved in reproductive health.

Hyperthyroidism:

Thyroid Overactivity: Hyperthyroidism is caused by an overproduction of thyroid hormones. This can result in symptoms such as weight loss, a racing heart, and anxiety.

Influence on Other Hormones:

Elevated thyroid hormone levels in women can disrupt the menstrual cycle, causing irregular periods or even amenorrhea (lack of menstruation). It can also have an effect on the balance of sex hormones.

Hormones of Reproduction:

Thyroid disease can cause menstrual irregularities by altering the production and control of reproductive hormones such as estrogen and progesterone.

Fertility Problems:

Both hypothyroidism and hyperthyroidism can impair fertility in men and women, making it difficult for couples to conceive.

The Adrenal Glands:

Thyroid hormones interact with the adrenal glands, which create cortisol, a stress hormone. Thyroid hormone imbalances can impact cortisol levels, contributing to conditions such as adrenal fatigue.

Insulin and Metabolism:

Thyroid hormones serve an important function in controlling metabolism. An imbalance can affect how the body absorbs nutrition and energy, which can contribute to weight gain or reduction. Thyroid dysfunction may also influence insulin sensitivity, contributing to issues such as insulin resistance.

Harmony of the Endocrine System:

The endocrine system is extremely linked, and perturbations in one component of the system can have an impact on others. Thyroid disorder can have an effect on the delicate balance of hormones in the body.

Insulin Resistance

Insulin resistance is a condition in which the body's cells become less sensitive to the effects of insulin, a hormone that regulates blood sugar (glucose) levels. While insulin resistance is most commonly connected with metabolic disorders like type 2 diabetes, it can also have an impact on hormonal balance.

Insulin not only regulates glucose levels, but it also interacts with other hormones in the body. Insulin resistance can cause abnormalities in these hormonal pathways, which contribute to imbalances. Here are some examples of how insulin resistance might disrupt hormonal balance:

- **Increased Insulin Levels:** The pancreas frequently generates more insulin in an attempt to overcome resistance. Elevated insulin levels can have an effect on other hormonal systems, potentially causing disturbances.

- **Sex Hormone Impact:** Insulin resistance has been linked to changes in sex hormone levels. It may contribute to greater levels of androgens (male hormones) in women, disrupting the regular menstrual cycle and leading to disorders like polycystic ovarian syndrome (PCOS). It can have an effect on testosterone levels in men.

- **Imbalance of Leptin and Ghrelin:** Insulin resistance can affect the balance of the hormones leptin and ghrelin, which regulate appetite and energy balance. This can exacerbate problems such as obesity and metabolic syndrome.

- **Cortisol Dysregulation:** Insulin and cortisol, a stress hormone, play important roles in blood sugar regulation. Insulin resistance may interfere with the normal cortisol response, thereby increasing stress and aggravating insulin resistance.

- Insulin resistance is connected with chronic low-grade inflammation and cytokines. This inflammatory condition can affect the synthesis

and action of several immune-related cytokines
and hormones.

- **Thyroid Dysfunction:** Some research suggests
  that insulin resistance and thyroid dysfunction
  are linked. Insulin resistance may impair thyroid
  hormone conversion, affecting total thyroid
  function.

Adrenal Fatigue

- Adrenal fatigue is a term used to describe a
  collection of nonspecific symptoms such as
  exhaustion, body aches, and anxiousness that are
  attributed to prolonged stress and a claimed
  adrenal gland failure. However, it is crucial to
  highlight that the concept of adrenal exhaustion
  is not universally acknowledged within the
  medical profession, and some specialists
  contend that there is insufficient scientific
  evidence to support it.

- By releasing chemicals such as cortisol and
  adrenaline, the adrenal glands, which are

positioned on top of each kidney, play an important part in the body's stress response. These hormones assist the body in responding effectively during times of extreme stress. Adrena exhaustion theory proposes that persistent stress can overstimulate the adrenal glands, eventually causing them to "burn out" and stop producing enough hormones, resulting in a range of symptoms.

- While persistent stress can have harmful effects on the body, the medical establishment is skeptical of the concept of adrenal exhaustion. Adrenal tiredness symptoms are widespread and can be suggestive of a variety of medical issues. Furthermore, laboratory studies for cortisol levels do not always support the diagnosis of adrenal fatigue.

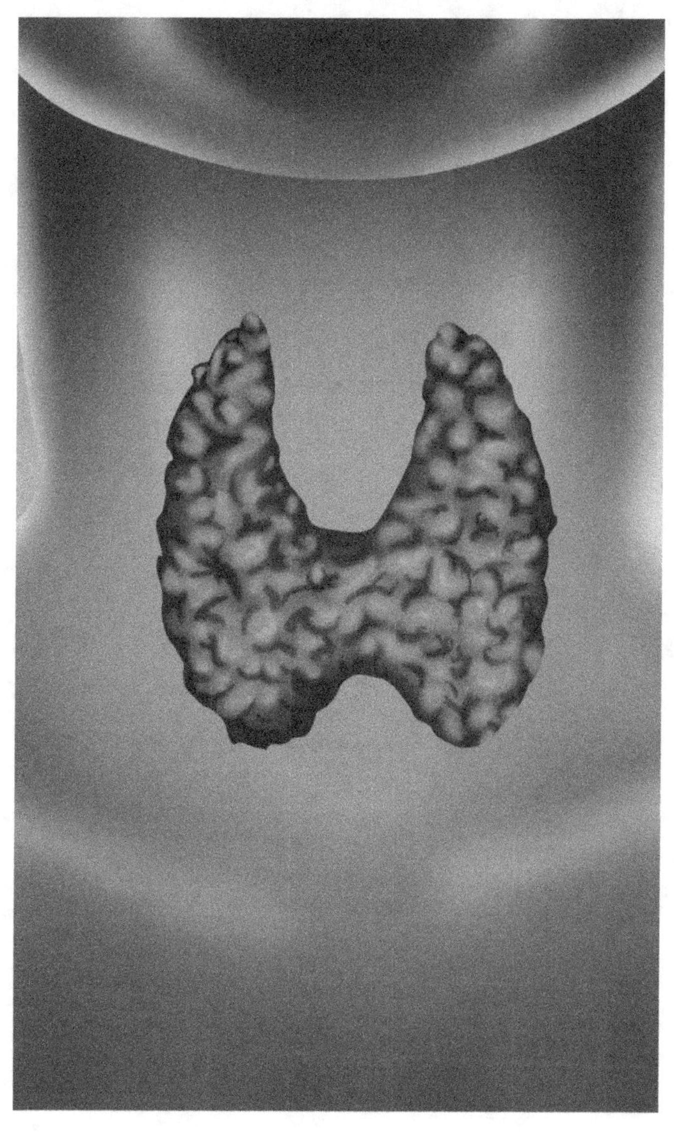

CHAPTER 4: LIFESTYLE AND HORMONAL HEALTH

The Impact of Diet

Blood Sugar Levels Are Balanced: A well-planned diet helps manage blood sugar levels, reducing insulin spikes and crashes. This is critical for hormonal balance, especially when dealing with insulin resistance.

- Essential Fatty Acids for Hormone Production: Essential fatty acids, such as omega-3 and omega-6, play an important role in hormone production. Included sources such as avocados, nuts, and fatty fish aid in hormone synthesis.

- Protein as a Building Block for Hormone Synthesis: Proteins serve as the building blocks for hormones. Adequate protein consumption aids in the production of hormones such as insulin and growth hormone.

Fiber for Gut Health: A high-fiber diet maintains a healthy gut microbiota, which influences hormone balance. A healthy stomach promotes adequate estrogen metabolism and overall hormonal balance.

Limiting Processed Foods:
Additives and preservatives in processed foods can affect endocrine function. Exposure to these disruptors is reduced by eating full, natural foods.

Managing Cortisol Levels with Vitamin C: Vitamin C aids in the management of cortisol, the stress hormone. Citrus fruits and bell peppers, for example, can help with stress resilience.

Zinc for Testosterone Production:

Zinc is required for testosterone production. Oysters, nuts, and seeds help to maintain adequate zinc levels, which benefits hormonal balance.

Magnesium for Sleep and Stress: Magnesium aids in relaxation and sleep quality, regulating hormone control indirectly. Magnesium-rich foods include leafy greens and almonds.

Foods that are anti-inflammatory: Chronic inflammation can affect hormone balance. Inflammation can be reduced by eating anti-inflammatory foods like turmeric, berries, and fatty fish.

Avoiding Excessive Caffeine:
While moderate caffeine consumption may be beneficial, excessive consumption might result in higher cortisol levels. Caffeine balance promotes hormonal wellness.

Endocrine Function and Vitamin D: Adequate vitamin D is essential for general endocrine function. Sunlight and vitamin D-rich foods like fatty fish and fortified dairy help to maintain hormonal equilibrium.

Iodine for Thyroid Health:

- Iodine is required for the generation of thyroid hormones. Iodine-rich foods, such as seaweed and iodized salt, help thyroid function.

- Cruciferous vegetables have chemicals that assist regulate estrogen levels, which is beneficial in conditions such as estrogen dominance. Broccoli, cabbage, and kale are some examples.

Maintaining a Healthy Body Weight:

Excess body weight, particularly visceral fat, can exacerbate hormone imbalances. A healthy weight is supported by a well-balanced diet and regular exercise.

Hydration for Hormonal transfer:

Proper hydration is required for hormone transfer throughout the body. Water promotes the proper functioning of the endocrine system.

Consumption of Nutrients:

Proteins:

Amino acids from protein-rich diets are required for hormone synthesis. Protein is required for the production of hormones such as insulin, growth hormone, and different neurotransmitters.

Fats:

Omega-3 fatty acids, for example, are precursors to hormones such as prostaglandins, which are implicated in inflammation and blood clotting. Saturated and trans fats may have an adverse effect on hormone production and function.

Carbohydrates:

Insulin levels can be influenced by the type and quality of carbohydrates consumed. Diets heavy in refined sugars and carbs may cause insulin resistance, altering blood sugar-regulating hormones

Fiber:

High-fiber diets can aid in blood sugar regulation and insulin sensitivity. This, in turn, has a favorable effect on hormones involved in metabolism.

Minerals and vitamins:

Vitamin D, zinc, magnesium, and other micronutrients are essential for hormone synthesis and activity. These vitamin deficiencies can alter hormonal equilibrium.

Hormone-Related Effects:

Insulin resistance can be exacerbated by a diet high in processed sugars and carbs. A well-balanced diet rich in complex carbs, fiber, and protein can help maintain insulin sensitivity.

Cortisol:

In addition to diet, chronic stress and lack of sleep also have an effect on cortisol levels. Balanced nutrition, stress management, and adequate sleep all contribute to optimal cortisol regulation.

Estrogen and testosterone:

Some foods include phytoestrogens, or chemicals that can affect estrogen levels. Similarly, zinc and vitamin D-rich foods can help maintain healthy testosterone levels.

Digestive Health:

The gut microbiome influences hormone metabolism and regulation. A high-fiber, fermented-food diet helps foster a healthy gut flora, which can improve hormonal balance.

Hydration:

Dehydration can have an impact on hormone synthesis and secretion. Hydration is critical for overall health, including hormone balance.

Caloric Consumption and Body

Composition:

Extreme caloric deficiencies or excesses can throw off hormonal balance, especially reproductive hormones.

Maintaining a healthy body composition with a well-balanced diet benefits hormonal health.

Foods to Avoid

- Processed foods contain refined sugars, artificial additives, and preservatives, which can disturb hormonal balance. Many packaged snacks, sugary beverages, and convenience foods fall under this category.
- Some doctors advise minimizing soy consumption since it includes chemicals that may mimic estrogen in the body. This could disrupt hormonal balance, especially in people who are sensitive to estrogen-like chemicals.
- Dairy: Some people are allergic to dairy, which causes inflammation and disrupts hormonal balance. Furthermore, many dairy products may contain hormones administered to cows, which might interfere with human hormonal levels.
- While moderate caffeine consumption is generally regarded as harmless, excessive consumption might result in increased cortisol levels, the stress hormone. Cortisol levels that

are too high can interfere with other hormone activities.

- Excessive alcohol consumption can impair the liver's ability to process hormones, resulting in hormonal abnormalities. It can also have an effect on sleep, which is essential for hormonal control.

- Trans Fats: Trans fats, which are found in many processed and fried meals, can contribute to inflammation and insulin resistance, affecting hormonal health.

- Foods with a high glycemic index: Foods that quickly boost blood sugar levels can cause insulin spikes. High insulin levels can interfere with hormonal balance and contribute to disorders such as insulin resistance.

- Artificial Sweeteners: According to some research, artificial sweeteners may disturb the gut microbiota, hence compromising hormonal balance. It is recommended that you eat these sweeteners in moderation.

- Non-organic Produce: Non-organic produce pesticides may include endocrine disrupting substances. Choosing organic fruits and vegetables can help decrease your exposure to these toxins.

- Excessive Red Meat: While lean and organic red meat can be part of a healthy diet, excessive consumption can lead to hormonal abnormalities. It is advised to diversify protein sources and incorporate plant-based options.

Exercise and Hormonal Balance

- Exercise is essential for maintaining hormonal balance and contributes greatly to what is commonly referred to as a "hormone fix." Hormones are chemical messengers that govern several physiological processes in the body, such as metabolism, mood, sleep, and reproduction. Regular physical activity can have a good impact on hormone production and balance, boosting general health and well-being.
- Insulin is a crucial hormone that is altered by exercise. Regular physical activity enhances insulin sensitivity, allowing for more effective blood sugar regulation. This is especially crucial in the prevention and management of disorders

like insulin resistance and type 2 diabetes. Furthermore, exercise helps reduce cortisol levels, a stress hormone. Chronic cortisol increase can cause a number of health concerns, including weight gain, immunological suppression, and cardiovascular problems. Individuals can manage stress and contribute to a more balanced cortisol level by engaging in regular exercise.

- Endorphins, also known as "feel-good" hormones, are produced during exercise. These neurotransmitters function as natural painkillers and mood lifters, promoting a sense of well-being and reducing pain perception. Regular physical activity has been related to improved mood and a reduction in anxiety and depression symptoms.

- Hormonal equilibrium is especially crucial for women at various phases of life. Regular exercise can help regulate menstrual cycles and decrease premenstrual syndrome (PMS) symptoms. Exercise helps alleviate some of the symptoms of menopause by lowering hot flashes and enhancing mood through the production of endorphins.

- Strength training in particular has been demonstrated to boost growth hormone production. Growth hormone is required for muscular development, fat metabolism, and anti-aging properties. Individuals can maintain hormonal balance and improve overall health by including resistance training into their workout program.

- Exercise helps to maintain a healthy body weight in addition to the direct impacts on various hormones. Excess body fat, particularly around the abdomen, has been linked to hormonal abnormalities such as increased insulin resistance and estrogen levels. Regular physical exercise aids in the regulation of body weight and composition, resulting in a healthy hormonal profile.

- It's crucial to remember that the type, intensity, and duration of exercise can all have an impact on hormone reactions. While moderate and consistent exercise is generally beneficial, excessive or vigorous activity without enough recovery may result in hormone imbalances. Balanced exercise, including aerobic, strength training, and flexibility activities, is essential for getting a complete hormone fix.

Finding the Right Balance

Hormone balance is critical for overall health and well-being. Obtaining the proper balance necessitates a combination of lifestyle decisions, food habits, and, in some situations, medical interventions. Here are some broad guidelines for establishing the proper hormonal balance:

- Dietary Guidelines:Consume a well-balanced diet that includes fruits, vegetables, whole grains, and lean proteins.
- Include healthy fats like omega-3 fatty acids from fish, flaxseeds, and walnuts.
- Limit your intake of processed meals, refined sugars, and caffeine.

- Exercise on a regular basis:Exercise on a regular basis, since it can help balance hormone levels and reduce stress.

- Aim for a combination of cardiovascular, strength, and flexibility workouts.

- A good night's sleep:Make sure you get enough rest each night. Sleep deprivation can affect hormone equilibrium.
- Create a soothing evening routine and stick to a consistent sleep schedule.

- Stress Reduction:Meditation, deep breathing, yoga, or mindfulness are all stress-reduction practices.
- Chronic stress can contribute to hormone abnormalities, so learning good stress management techniques is critical.

- Hydration:Stay hydrated since water is necessary for many biological activities, including hormone control.

- Toxins Should Be Avoided:Reduce your exposure to environmental pollutants and endocrine disruptors found in certain plastics, insecticides, and household items.

- Limit your intake of alcohol and caffeine:Excessive alcohol and caffeine use can have an effect on hormone levels. Consume these ingredients in moderation.

- Keep a Healthy Weight:It is critical for hormonal balance to achieve and maintain a healthy weight. Excess body fat, particularly around the belly, can interfere with hormone synthesis.

- Regular Health Examinations:Schedule regular check-ups with your doctor to monitor hormone levels and correct any imbalances.

- Consider Getting Professional Advice:Consult a healthcare practitioner if you suspect a hormone imbalance or are experiencing symptoms. They can administer tests and make tailored recommendations or actions.

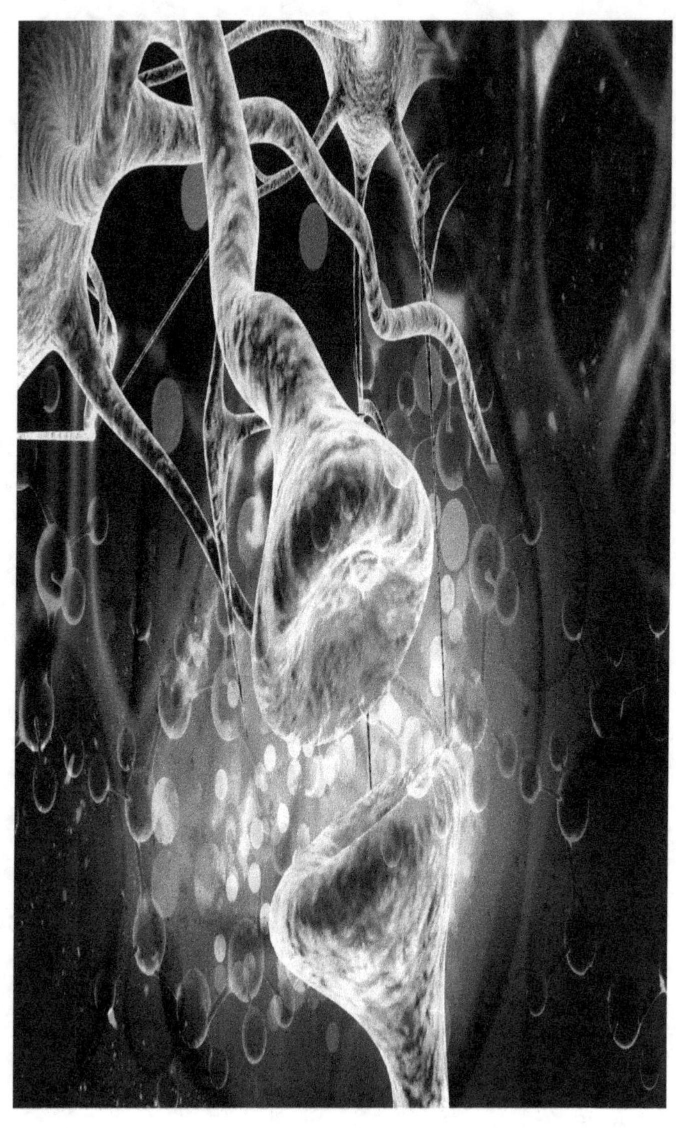

CHAPTER 5: NATURAL REMEDIES AND SUPPLEMENTS

Herbal Support

The following herbs are frequently referenced in the context of hormonal support;

This adaptogenic herb (Withania somnifera): Is known to help balance cortisol levels, potentially promoting overall hormonal balance.

Maca (Lepidium meyenii): Maca is well-known for its ability to support hormone balance, notably in the endocrine system.

Vitex (Vitex agnus-castus): Also known as chasteberry, vitex is said to affect hormonal balance, particularly during the menstrual cycle.

Actaea racemosa (Black Cohosh): Native Americans have traditionally employed black cohosh to help with hormonal balance, particularly in menopausal women.

Dong Quai (Angelica sinensis): In Traditional Chinese Medicine, dong quai is thought to support hormonal balance, particularly in the female reproductive system.

Rhodiola (Rhodiola rosea): This adaptogenic plant may aid in stress adaptation by modulating hormone responses.

Licorice Root (Glycyrrhiza glabra): It is thought that licorice root affects cortisol levels, potentially altering overall hormonal balance.

Holy Basil (Ocimum sanctum): Also known as tulsi, holy basil is an adaptogen that may help the body cope with stress by influencing hormonal responses.

Red Clover (Trifolium pratense): Red clover includes isoflavones, which have estrogen-like actions and may alter hormonal balance.

Saw Palmetto (Serenoa repens): Saw palmetto is frequently related with male prostate health and may alter hormonal balance.

Essential Nutrients

Fatty Acids Omega-3:

- Fatty fish (salmon, mackerel, sardines), flaxseeds, chia seeds, and walnuts contain it.
- Omega-3 fatty acids promote hormone synthesis and minimize inflammation.

D vitamin:

- Sunlight, fatty fish, fortified dairy products, and supplements are all sources of vitamin D.
- Essential for hormonal balance, including insulin and sex hormone regulation.

B6 vitamin:

- Poultry, seafood, bananas, avocados, and fortified cereals all contain it.
- Helps to produce neurotransmitters and hormones such as serotonin and melatonin.

E vitamin:

- Nuts, seeds, spinach, and broccoli all contain it.

- As an antioxidant, it aids in hormone homeostasis and the reduction of oxidative stress.

Magnesium:
- Green leafy vegetables, nuts, seeds, and whole grains all contain it.
- Aids in the function of the endocrine system and the regulation of cortisol levels.

Zinc:
- Obtained from the consumption of meat, seafood, legumes, and seeds.
- It is required for the generation and function of hormones such as insulin and thyroid hormones.

Iron:
- Lean meats, beans, and dark leafy greens are high in this nutrient.
- Supports overall energy levels and aids in the prevention of hormonal abnormalities associated with anemia.

Protein:

- Meat, fish, dairy, eggs, and plant-based alternatives like lentils and tofu are also good sources.
- It is necessary for the generation of hormones and aids in the stabilization of blood sugar levels.

Fiber:

- Fruits, vegetables, whole grains, and legumes contain it.
- Supports intestinal health, which might have an indirect effect on hormone balance.

Probiotics:

- Fermented foods such as yogurt, kefir, sauerkraut, and kimchi contain probiotics.
- Helps with intestinal health, which is linked to hormonal balance and overall well-being.

Iodine:

- Seaweed, salmon, dairy products, and iodized salt all contain iodine.
- Thyroid hormone synthesis, which regulates metabolism, is required.

Selenium:

- Brazil nuts, seafood, meat, and whole grains all contain it.
- Supports thyroid hormone conversion and protects against oxidative damage.

Minerals for Hormonal Health

- Zinc is required for the development and function of hormones such as insulin and sex hormones. It is also involved in thyroid hormone conversion. Oysters, steak, pumpkin seeds, and lentils are zinc-rich foods.
- Selenium is necessary for the creation of thyroid hormones, which control metabolism. Selenium is found in Brazil nuts, seafood, poultry, and whole grains.
- Iodine is required for the formation of thyroid hormones. Iodine is found in seafood, seaweed, dairy products, and iodized salt.
- Magnesium: Magnesium aids in the manufacture of sex hormones and the regulation of cortisol levels. Magnesium is abundant in leafy green vegetables, nuts, seeds, and whole grains.

- Copper is required for the creation of various hormones, including thyroid hormones and estrogen. Copper is found in foods such as organ meats, shellfish, nuts, and seeds.
- Iron: Iron is necessary for the delivery of oxygen in the blood and for the regulation of thyroid hormones. Iron-rich foods include lean meats, beans, lentils, and fortified cereals.
- Vitamin D: Although it is not a mineral, vitamin D is essential for hormonal equilibrium. It modulates the expression of genes involved in insulin synthesis and aids in the maintenance of sex hormone balance. Vitamin D is found in sunlight, fatty fish, and fortified meals.
- Calcium plays a function in the control of parathyroid hormone, which regulates calcium and phosphorus metabolism. Calcium is found in dairy products, leafy green vegetables, and fortified plant-based milk.

Hormone-Supporting Supplements

D vitamin:

Vitamin D, also known as the "sunshine vitamin," is essential for hormone production. It aids in the manufacture of hormones such as testosterone.

Fatty Acids Omega-3:

Omega-3 fatty acids, which can be found in fish oil, flaxseed oil, and walnuts, boost hormone production and reduce inflammation, which helps improve hormonal balance.

Magnesium:

Magnesium participates in nearly 300 physiological activities in the body, including hormone control. It's in nuts, seeds, and leafy green vegetables.

Zinc:

Zinc is present in meat, dairy, nuts, and seeds and is required for the creation of testosterone and other hormones. It is very critical for male reproductive health.

B6 vitamin:

This vitamin aids in the production of neurotransmitters and steroid hormones. Vitamin B6-rich foods include poultry, fish, potatoes, and fortified cereals.

Ashwagandha:

Ashwagandha, an adaptogenic plant, may help regulate cortisol levels, aiding the body's response to stress and perhaps influencing hormonal equilibrium.

Rosea Rhodiola:

Rhodiola Rosea is another adaptogenic herb that is thought to help the body adapt to stress and balance cortisol levels.

Root of Maca:

Maca is a Peruvian plant whose root is said to assist balance hormones, particularly in regard to reproductive health.

Diindolylmethane (DIM):

DIM, which is found in cruciferous vegetables such as broccoli, aids in the maintenance of a healthy estrogen balance in the body.

Vitex agnus-castus (Chaste Tree Berry):

Vitex is frequently used to improve hormonal balance in women, particularly during the menstrual cycle, by modulating pituitary gland activity.

Probiotics

Gut-Brain Axis:

The gut is often referred to as the "second brain" because to the gut-brain axis, which is a bidirectional communication connection between the central nervous system and the gastrointestinal tract. Probiotics may have an effect on this axis, influencing the release and control of specific hormones.

Estrogen Metabolism:

Some research has looked into the involvement of gut flora in estrogen metabolism. A healthy gut flora may help with estrogen metabolism, which is important for hormonal balance, especially in women.

Probiotics and Inflammation:

Probiotics may assist to modulate inflammation in the body. Chronic inflammation has the potential to impair hormonal homeostasis, particularly the stress hormone cortisol. Probiotics may indirectly contribute to hormonal balance by fostering a healthy inflammatory response.

Insulin Sensitivity:

Healthy insulin levels are essential for hormonal homeostasis. Some study suggests that probiotics may improve insulin sensitivity, presumably influencing blood sugar-regulating hormones.

Appetite Hormonal Regulation:

The gut microbiota can alter the production of peptides that govern appetite. Probiotics may indirectly contribute to hormonal regulation of hunger and satiety by supporting a healthy gut environment.

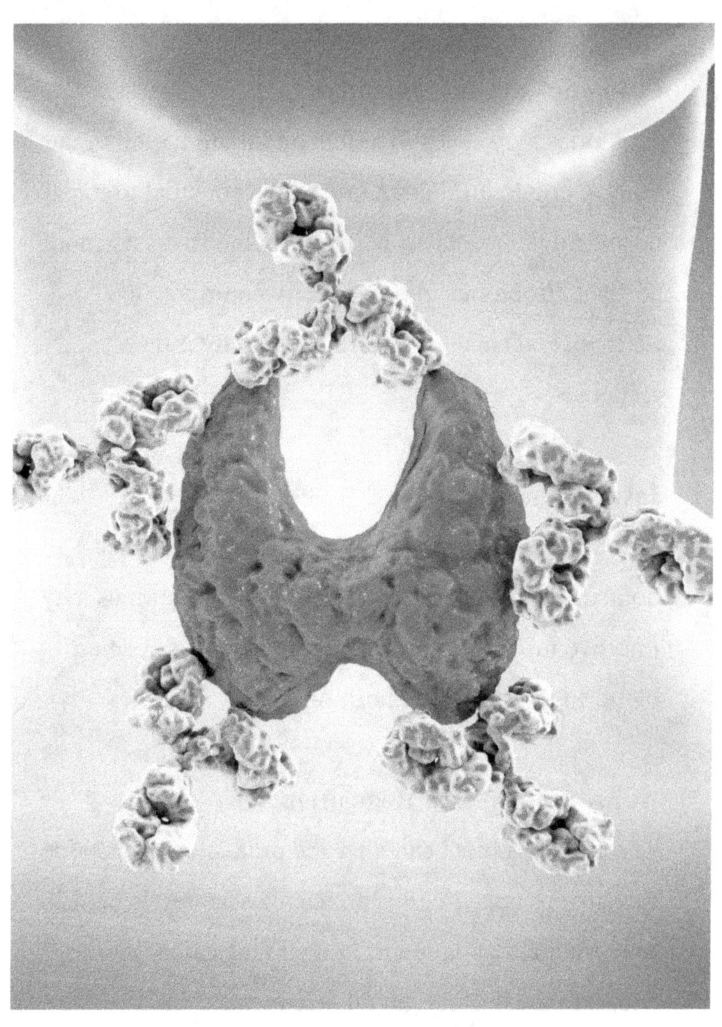

CHAPTER 6: LIFESTYLE CHANGES FOR HORMONE OPTIMIZATION

Stress Management Techniques

Stress management is essential for hormone optimization since prolonged stress can disturb hormone balance in the body, leading to a variety of health problems. Stress reduction and hormone balance can be achieved by incorporating lifestyle adjustments. Here are some stress management approaches that can be implemented as lifestyle modifications to optimize hormones:

Exercise on a regular basis:
Exercise on a regular basis, such as aerobics, yoga, or strength training.

Exercise causes the release of endorphins, which function as natural mood lifters and can impact hormone balance.

A good night's sleep:

Make it a point to get 7-9 hours of decent sleep each night.

Sleep deprivation can influence cortisol levels and insulin sensitivity, influencing hormone balance.

Nutrition that is well-balanced:

Consume a diet rich in fruits, vegetables, whole grains, and lean proteins.

Include omega-3 fatty acid-rich items in your diet since they can help control stress hormones.

Meditation and mindfulness:

Reduce tension and improve relaxation by practicing mindfulness meditation or deep breathing exercises.

Mindfulness can aid in the regulation of cortisol levels and the overall balance of hormones.

Social Interactions:

Make and keep strong social connections.

Spending time with loved ones and developing a support network can have a favorable impact on stress hormones.

Limit your intake of caffeine and sugar:
Reduce your intake of caffeine and sugary meals. Caffeine can increase cortisol production, and sugar increases can influence insulin levels.

Time Administration:
To efficiently manage time, prioritize work and create realistic goals.
Controlling your schedule might help you minimize stress and prevent hormone abnormalities.

Exposure to Nature:
Spend time in nature, whether it's a stroll around the park or a hike.
Exposure to nature has been related to lower cortisol levels and overall well-being.

Hobbies and recreational activities:
Engage in things that you enjoy to encourage relaxation and stress reduction.

Hobbies can be a terrific method to distract yourself from worries and promote hormonal balance.

Limit Your Screen Time:

Reduce screen time, especially before bedtime.

Blue light from screens can interrupt sleep patterns and interfere with hormone control.

Hydration:

Keep yourself hydrated by drinking plenty of water throughout the day.

Dehydration can cause stress in the body and disrupt hormone levels.

A Nutrient-Dense Diet

Hormone function optimization is critical for general health and well-being. A nutrient-dense diet can help support hormonal balance significantly. Here are some lifestyle and dietary adjustments that can help with hormone optimization:

1. Macronutrient Balance:

Include a variety of carbohydrates, proteins, and fats in your diet. Each macronutrient contributes to hormone production and control.

Avocados, olive oil, and almonds are high in healthy fats, which aid in hormone synthesis.

2. Protein-Rich Foods:

Protein is required for hormone production. Include lean meats, fish, eggs, beans, and plant-based proteins in your daily diet.

Adequate protein consumption promotes muscular health, which is related to hormonal balance.

3. A range of Colorful Fruits and Vegetables:

A range of colorful fruits and vegetables provide critical vitamins, minerals, and antioxidants.

Antioxidants aid in the fight against oxidative stress, which can affect hormonal homeostasis.

4. Whole Grains:

Whole grains are preferable to processed carbs. Whole grains are high in fiber, vitamins, and minerals, which promote general health.

Fiber aids in blood sugar regulation, which is essential for insulin sensitivity.

5. Omega-3 Fatty Acids:

Include omega-3 fatty acid sources such as fatty fish (salmon, mackerel), chia seeds, flaxseeds, and walnuts in your diet.
Omega-3 fatty acids promote brain health and can alter hormone production.

6. Vitamin D:

Make sure you get enough vitamin D, either from sunlight or food sources such fatty fish, fortified dairy, and pills if necessary.
Vitamin D is required for the creation of several hormones.

Minerals:

Zinc, magnesium, and selenium are minerals that are necessary for hormonal equilibrium. Include nuts, seeds, whole grains, and leafy green vegetables among your sources.
These minerals are essential for hormone synthesis and control.

8. Hydration:

Staying hydrated is important for overall health, including hormone balance.

Water aids in the passage of hormones through the bloodstream and aids in metabolic activities.

9. Limit Processed meals and Sugar:

Excessive sugar consumption and processed meals can cause insulin resistance and disturb hormone balance.

To lessen the danger of hormone abnormalities, eat full, unprocessed meals.

10. Regular Physical Activity:

Exercise improves hormonal balance by increasing insulin sensitivity and endorphin release.

Aim for a combination of aerobic, strength, and flexibility activities.

11. Adequate Sleep:

Make excellent sleep a priority because it is necessary for hormone control, particularly growth hormone and cortisol.

Establish a regular sleep pattern and practice good sleep hygiene.

12. Stress Management:
Chronic stress can wreak havoc on hormonal equilibrium. Incorporate stress-relieving activities like meditation, yoga, or deep breathing techniques. Make time in your schedule for rest and self-care.

13. Consult a Healthcare Professional: If you suspect hormone irregularities, get medical attention. They can administer tests and provide personalized advice.

Adequate Sleep

Adequate sleep is an important part of living a healthy lifestyle, and it plays an important role in hormone optimization. Hormones are chemical messengers that control many physiological processes in the body, such as metabolism, stress response, immunological function, and growth. Here's how getting enough sleep can help with hormone optimization:

Growth Hormone (GH) Secretion:

The majority of growth hormone is produced during deep sleep, particularly in the first half of the night. This hormone is necessary for growth, cell repair, and overall health.

Cortisol Control:

Sleep aids in the regulation of cortisol, the stress hormone. Chronic sleep loss can raise cortisol levels, which can contribute to stress, inflammation, and weight gain.

Sensitivity to Insulin:

Sleep deprivation is linked to insulin resistance, which can contribute to the development of type 2 diabetes. Adequate sleep aids in the maintenance of optimal insulin sensitivity, hence promoting overall metabolic health.

Balance of Leptin and Ghrelin:

Sleep deprivation can upset the balance of the chemicals leptin and ghrelin, which regulate hunger. Inadequate sleep frequently causes an increase in ghrelin (an appetite-stimulating hormone) and a reduction in leptin

(an appetite-suppressing hormone), both of which can
contribute to overeating and weight gain.

Thyroid Activity:

Sleep is essential for thyroid-stimulating hormone (TSH)
modulation and thyroid gland general function. Thyroid
health is critical for metabolism and energy balance.

Production of Testosterone and Estrogen:

In men, testosterone is mostly created when sleeping,
and a lack of sleep can result in reduced testosterone
levels. Proper sleep promotes healthy estrogen levels in
women. Imbalances in these sex hormones can have an
impact on mood, energy, and reproductive health.

Melatonin Synthesis:

Melatonin, the hormone that regulates sleep-wake
cycles, is generated during times of darkness. Adequate
sleep promotes better sleep quality by promoting a
healthy circadian rhythm and optimum melatonin
synthesis.

To optimize your hormones, incorporate appropriate sleep into your daily routine:
Sleep should be prioritized. 7-9 hours of quality sleep per night is recommended.

Create a Consistent Sleep Schedule: Go to bed and wake up at the same time every day, including weekends.

Create a Relaxing Bedtime Routine: Establish routines that tell your body it's time to unwind, such as reading, gently stretching, or having a warm bath.

Make Your Bedroom Sleep-Friendly: Make your bedroom sleep-friendly by keeping it dark, quiet, and at a pleasant temperature.

Limit Screen Time Before Bed: Limit your exposure to blue light from screens at least an hour before bedtime to support natural melatonin production.

Regular Exercise

Regular physical activity can have a substantial impact on hormone optimization. Hormones play an important part in many physiological functions, and exercise has been found to improve their production and balance. Here are several ways that regular exercise can help with hormone optimization:

- Regular physical exercise improves insulin sensitivity, allowing the body to use insulin more effectively. This can be especially helpful in avoiding and controlling illnesses such as type 2 diabetes. Insulin balance is beneficial to overall hormonal health.

- Exercise can aid in the regulation of cortisol, the stress hormone. While short-term cortisol rises during exercise are appropriate, longterm cortisol elevation owing to stress can be harmful. Regular physical activity, particularly yoga and moderate cardiovascular exercise, can aid in the management of stress and cortisol levels.

- **Growth Hormone Release:** High-intensity interval training (HIIT) and resistance training both stimulate the release of growth hormone. This hormone is required for cell development, repair, and metabolism. Adequate growth hormone levels help to keep muscular mass and fat at bay.

- Resistance training, in particular, has been associated to an increase in testosterone production. Testosterone is necessary for muscular growth, bone health, and general vitality. A regular strength training practice can help to maintain healthy testosterone levels.

- **Thyroid Function:** Exercise can improve thyroid function, which is necessary for metabolism regulation. Aerobic and resistance training may both help to maintain a healthy thyroid hormone balance.

- Regular physical activity can aid in the regulation of appetite hormones such as leptin and ghrelin. This can help with weight management by suppressing hunger and encouraging a healthy balance of calorie intake and expenditure.

- **Endorphin Release:** Exercise causes the release of endorphins, sometimes known as "feel-good" hormones. These hormones not only contribute to a good mood, but they also help with pain and stress management.

- **Menstrual Cycle Regularity:** In women, regular exercise can help with menstrual cycle regularity. Excessive activity, especially when mixed with low body fat, can cause menstruation irregularities, so finding a happy medium is essential.

Detoxification Strategies

Detoxification techniques can help to optimize hormone balance and promote general well-being. Here are some lifestyle adjustments that can help with hormone optimization via detoxification:

Eating Well:

To decrease your exposure to pesticides and chemicals, choose organic, complete foods.

Include plenty of fruits and vegetables to acquire the vitamins, minerals, and antioxidants you need to assist your detoxification pathways.

Hydration:

Maintain enough hydration to aid in the removal of toxins through urine.

Consider including herbal drinks recognized for their detoxifying effects, such as dandelion or green tea.

Reduce your intake of processed foods:

Reduce your intake of processed foods, which frequently contain additives, preservatives, and artificial chemicals that can interfere with hormone balance.

Limit your intake of sugar and caffeine:

Reduce your intake of processed sweets and caffeine, as they might lead to hormonal imbalances and liver damage.

Macronutrients in Balance:
To boost energy levels and hormone production, consume a balanced diet of carbohydrates, proteins, and healthy fats.

Diet High in Fiber:
Include fiber-rich foods like whole grains, legumes, and vegetables to promote regular bowel movements and toxin disposal.

Exercise on a regular basis:
Exercise on a daily basis to assist circulation and the lymphatic system, which aids in the removal of toxins from the body.

Sauna Treatment:
Saunas can cause perspiration, which aids in toxin clearance through the skin. This can help with general detoxification.

A good night's sleep:

Make quality sleep a priority to allow the body to recover and replenish. Sleep is essential for maintaining hormonal balance and overall wellness.

Stress Reduction:

Hormone levels might be affected by chronic stress. Incorporate stress-relieving methods into your everyday routine, such as meditation, deep breathing, yoga, or mindfulness.

Herbs and supplements:

Consider liver-supporting vitamins and herbs such as milk thistle, dandelion root, and turmeric. Before incorporating new supplements into your routine, consult with a healthcare practitioner.

Toxin Awareness in the Environment:

Environmental contaminants in personal care items, household cleaners, and plastics should be avoided. Choose natural and environmentally beneficial options.

Detox Periods on a Regular Basis:

To support the body's natural detoxification processes, implement periodic detox procedures under the supervision of a healthcare expert.

Hormone-Friendly Supplements

Breakfast Boosters

Protein-rich foods include:

Protein-rich foods include eggs, Greek yogurt, and lean meats. Protein aids in hormone production and can keep you feeling full and pleased.

Fats that are good for you:

Avocado, nuts, and seeds are high in good fats, which are required for hormone production. Omega-3 fatty acids, which are found in fatty fish such as salmon and chia seeds, are very useful.

Fiber:

Whole grains, fruits, and vegetables include fiber, which can help to keep blood sugar levels stable. Blood sugar control is critical for hormonal balance.

Berries:

Berries are high in antioxidants, which can assist the body fight oxidative stress. This may have a beneficial effect on hormonal balance.

Tea, green:

Green tea contains antioxidants and chemicals that may benefit hormone balances. It also gives you a light caffeine rush.

Greens with leaves:

Spinach, kale, and other leafy greens are high in vitamins and minerals, which promote general health and hormone function.

Chia seeds

Chia seeds contain omega-3 fatty acids, fiber, and protein. They go well with yogurt, smoothies, and cereal.

Turmeric:

Curcumin, the main ingredient in turmeric, is anti-inflammatory and may help with hormonal balance.

Cinnamon:

Cinnamon can aid in the regulation of blood sugar levels, which is essential for hormonal health.

Yogurt fortified with probiotics:
Probiotics, which are included in some yogurts, may improve intestinal health, which in turn might affect hormone balance

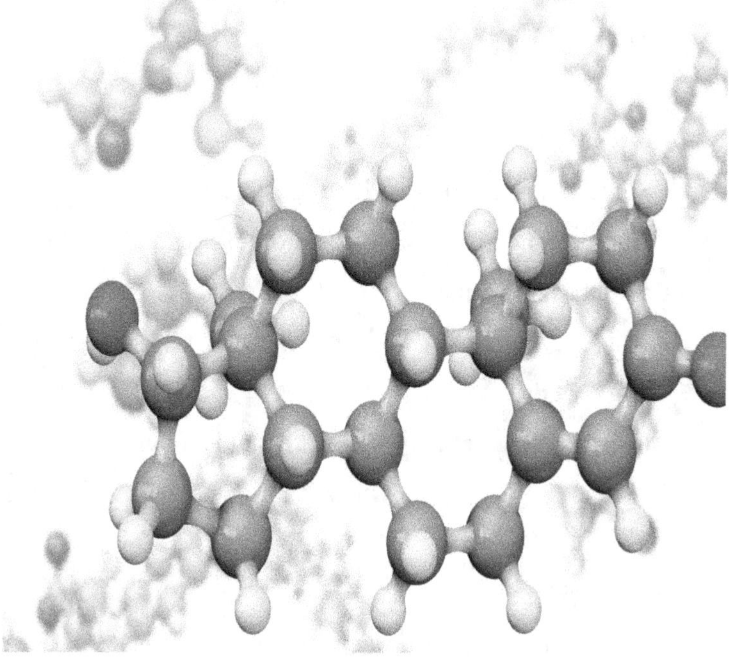

CHAPTER 6: TARGETED TREATMENTS FOR SPECIFIC HORMONAL IMBALANCES

Natural Therapies for Estrogen Dominance

Dietary Modifications:

- Cruciferous Vegetables: Foods like broccoli, cauliflower, kale, and Brussels sprouts contain estrogen-metabolizing chemicals.
- Whole grains, fruits, and vegetables high in fiber can aid in the removal of excess estrogen from the body.

Supplements:

- DIM (Diindolylmethane): Found in cruciferous vegetables, DIM aids in estrogen metabolism.

- Calcium D-Glucarate: This supplement may aid in the elimination of excess estrogen in the body.

Herbal Treatments:

- Chasteberry (Vitex): Known for its capacity to balance hormones, chasteberry can aid in menstrual cycle regulation and alleviate symptoms of estrogen dominance.
- Milk Thistle: Aids liver function, which is required for hormone metabolization, especially estrogen.
- Turmeric has anti-inflammatory qualities and may aid with estrogen regulation.

Fats that are good for you:

Omega-3 fatty acid sources, such as flaxseeds, chia seeds, and fatty fish, may help balance hormones.

Stress Management:

Hormonal imbalances can be exacerbated by chronic stress. Yoga, meditation, and deep breathing are all practices that can help you manage your stress.

Exercise:

Regular physical exercise promotes overall hormonal balance and can aid in weight management, both of which are essential for estrogen balance.

Avoid Hormone Disruptors:

Reduce your exposure to endocrine disruptors and environmental contaminants found in certain plastics, personal care items, and pesticides.

Keep a Healthy Weight:

Estrogen can be produced and stored by fat cells. Maintaining a healthy weight through diet and exercise can aid with hormone regulation.

A Healthy Way of Life:

As insufficient sleep can alter hormone balance, get appropriate sleep and develop a regular sleep routine.

Testosterone Replacement Therapy for Men

TRT is a medical intervention that aims to restore testosterone levels in men who have low or insufficient levels of this vital hormone. Testosterone is a vital hormone that promotes secondary sexual traits such as muscular mass, bone density, and facial hair, as well as the development and maintenance of male reproductive tissues.

Here are some important considerations to consider while considering Testosterone Replacement Therapy:

TRT indications include:

Low Testosterone Levels: TRT is often prescribed for men who have clinically low testosterone levels, as shown by blood tests. Low testosterone symptoms may include fatigue, decreased libido, erectile dysfunction, depression, and poor cognitive function.

TRT comes in several varieties.

Injections: Testosterone can be delivered intramuscularly, often once every one to two weeks. This is a standard approach that allows for consistent hormone release.

Topical Gels or Patches: Some TRT methods include applying testosterone gels or patches to the skin. These are absorbed into the bloodstream, allowing for controlled hormone release.

Testosterone pellets are tiny, subcutaneous implants that are implanted beneath the skin. They produce a steady amount of testosterone over a period of months.

Regular Blood Tests: Patients undergoing TRT should have their testosterone levels checked on a regular basis by blood tests. This verifies that the medication is working and that testosterone levels are within the normal range.

Dosage Adjustments: The dosage of testosterone may be changed to achieve ideal levels based on the monitoring findings and the patient's response.

Potential Advantages: more Energy and Mood: Many men report more energy, improved mood, and a sense of well-being after receiving TRT.

Muscle Mass and Bone Density: Testosterone is essential for sustaining muscle mass and bone density. TRT may help to improve these conditions.

Enhanced Libido and Sexual performance: Testosterone is essential for sexual health, and TRT may assist men with low testosterone increase their libido and erectile performance.

Considerations and risks: TRT has the potential for adverse effects such as acne, fluid retention, and alterations in cholesterol levels. Patients must discuss these potential concerns with their healthcare professional.

Prostate Health Monitoring: There is continuing study into the potential impact of TRT on prostate health. Regular monitoring is essential, including prostate-specific antigen (PSA) tests.

Individual Response: Individual responses to TRT can differ. Some men may see major gains, while others may see just minor improvements.

Thyroid Hormone Replacement Therapy

- Thyroid hormone replacement therapy is a common medical treatment for thyroid problems such as hypothyroidism. The thyroid gland, located in the neck, generates hormones (thyroxine or T4 and triiodothyronine or T3) that regulate metabolism, energy production, and other physiological activities.

- Hypothyroidism occurs when the thyroid gland does not generate enough thyroid hormones, resulting in fatigue, weight gain, cold sensitivity, and sadness. In such circumstances, thyroid hormone replacement treatment is suggested to supplement or replace the insufficient thyroid hormone production.

- Synthetic thyroxine (levothyroxine), which is similar to the T4 hormone naturally produced by the thyroid gland, is the most often used drug for thyroid hormone replacement. Levothyroxine is often taken orally and aids in the restoration of normal thyroid hormone levels in the body.

- Thyroid hormone replacement therapy aims to alleviate hypothyroidism symptoms, restore thyroid hormone levels in the blood, and preserve overall health. The medicine dosage is carefully adjusted based on the patient's age, weight, and the severity of their thyroid malfunction. Thyroid hormone levels must be monitored on a regular basis by blood tests to ensure that the dosage remains suitable.

- Individuals having thyroid hormone replacement therapy must carefully follow their healthcare provider's recommendations, take the medication on a consistent basis, and attend regular follow-up sessions. Dosage adjustments may be required over time, and healthcare experts may also examine other factors, such as the existence of other medical problems or drugs that may impair thyroid function.

Insulin-Sensitizing Medications

Insulin-sensitizing pharmaceuticals are a type of prescription that helps increase the body's responsiveness to insulin, a hormone that regulates blood sugar (glucose) levels. These drugs are widely used to treat illnesses like type 2 diabetes, where insulin resistance is a major role.

The following are some of the most common insulin-sensitizing medications:

Metformin:

- Metformin works largely by decreasing glucose synthesis in the liver and increasing insulin sensitivity in peripheral tissues such as muscles.
- It is frequently used as the first-line treatment for type 2 diabetes. Metformin can also help with weight loss and cardiovascular health.

Thiazolidinediones (TZDs, sometimes known as glitazones):

- Rosiglitazone and pioglitazone are two examples.
- TZDs work by activating peroxisome proliferator-activated receptor gamma

(PPAR-gamma), a nuclear receptor that controls gene expression. As a result, insulin sensitivity improves in adipose tissue, skeletal muscle, and the liver.

- Benefits: Although TZDs are successful at reducing insulin resistance, they may cause weight gain and fluid retention.

Agonists of the GLP-1 Receptor:

- Exenatide, liraglutide, and dulaglutide are a few examples.
- Action Mechanism: GLP-1 receptor agonists enhance insulin secretion, decrease glucagon secretion, slow stomach emptying, and increase satiety. They improve insulin sensitivity indirectly.
- GLP-1 receptor agonists may contribute to weight loss and have cardiovascular advantages in addition to their glucose-lowering effects.

Inhibitors of SGLT-2:

- Canagliflozin, dapagliflozin, and empagliflozin are a few examples.

- Sodium-glucose co-transporter 2 (SGLT-2) inhibitors decrease glucose reabsorption in the kidneys, resulting in increased glucose excretion in the urine. This enhances insulin sensitivity indirectly.

- Benefits: SGLT-2 inhibitors provide cardiovascular and renal benefits in addition to lowering blood glucose levels. They may also contribute to weight loss.

Adrenal Support Supplements

Vitamin C: Is necessary for adrenal function and is frequently included in adrenal support supplements due to its antioxidant effects.

B vitamins, particularly B5 (pantothenic acid) and B6, are essential for adrenal function and stress hormone synthesis.

Magnesium: This mineral is involved in a variety of physiological functions, including stress response.

Herbs that assist the body adapt to stress are known as adaptogens. Among the most common adaptogens discovered in adrenal support supplements are:

- **Rhodiola Rosea**: This herb is said to boost the body's tolerance to stress.
- Ashwagandha is well-known for its ability to alleviate stress and anxiety.
- **Tulsi (Holy Basil):** Used traditionally for its anti-stress effects.
- **Licorice Root:** This herb is known to support adrenal function and may help keep cortisol levels in check.

Vitamin D levels are vital for overall health, and some research imply a link between vitamin D insufficiency and adrenal difficulties.

Zinc: An vital mineral that aids immunological function and may be found in adrenal support formulas.

Omega-3 Fatty Acids: These fatty acids, found in fish oil, have anti-inflammatory qualities and may benefit overall health, including adrenal function.

CHAPTER 7: SPECIAL CONSIDERATIONS FOR WOMEN AND MEN

Women's Hormonal Health

The Menstrual Cycle and Reproductive Hormones:
The menstrual cycle is an important element of a woman's hormonal health. It is controlled by a careful balance of hormones that includes estrogen and progesterone. These hormones are in charge of uterine lining formation, ovulation, and preparing the body for a possible pregnancy. Hormone imbalances can cause irregular menstruation periods, fertility difficulties, and other reproductive health issues.

Puberty and Adolescence:
The journey from childhood to adulthood is marked by hormonal changes throughout puberty. Hormonal changes, notably estrogen, influence the onset of menstruation, breast development, and the growth of

pubic and underarm hair. Understanding and regulating these changes is critical for young women's physical and mental well-being.

Pregnancy and Hormonal Changes:
A healthy pregnancy requires considerable hormonal alterations to promote fetal development. Human chorionic gonadotropin (hCG), progesterone, and estrogen all play important roles in pregnancy maintenance, fetal growth, and preparing the body for labor and lactation.

Menopause and Hormonal Transition: Menopause is the end of a woman's reproductive years, which commonly occurs in her late 40s or early 50s. The production of estrogen and progesterone decreases throughout menopause, resulting in a variety of physical and emotional changes. Hot flashes, mood swings, and changes in bone density are all possible symptoms. Hormone replacement therapy (HRT) may be used to ease these symptoms in some cases, but it is not without hazards, and individual considerations are critical.

Hormonal problems and Health Conditions:

A variety of hormonal problems can have an impact on a woman's health. Polycystic ovarian syndrome (PCOS), for example, is characterized by a hormonal imbalance that can result in irregular periods, fertility concerns, and metabolic challenges. Endometriosis is another illness that causes pain and infertility by causing tissue to develop outside the uterus.

Hormones and Mental Health:

Hormonal variations can have an impact on one's mood and mental health. Premenstrual syndrome (PMS), for example, is a mix of physical and emotional symptoms that occur prior to menstruation. Pregnancy and the postpartum period are also linked to mood disorders like postpartum depression.

Maintaining Hormonal Balance:

Lifestyle factors such as nutrition, exercise, and stress management all have a part in hormonal balance. Regular exercise, a nutritious diet, and stress-reduction tactics can all help to improve hormonal health.

Hormonal Balance During Menopause

- Menopause is a natural biological process that occurs when a woman's reproductive years come to an end. It is described as the lack of menstrual cycles for 12 consecutive months and often happens in the late 40s or early 50s. One of the most important parts of menopause is the hormonal changes that occur in a woman's body, which cause a variety of physical and emotional symptoms.

- The ovaries generate estrogen and progesterone, which are the key hormones implicated in menopause. The ovaries gradually generate less of these hormones as a woman approaches menopause, resulting in hormonal oscillations and imbalances. This drop in hormone levels can cause a variety of symptoms, including hot flashes, nocturnal sweats, mood swings, and sleep pattern abnormalities.

- Estrogen, in particular, is essential for regulating the menstrual cycle and maintaining the health of reproductive tissues such as the breasts, uterus, and vagina. The decrease in estrogen during menopause can cause symptoms such as vaginal dryness, libido loss, and an increased risk of osteoporosis.

- Hormonal balancing is a complex and dynamic process throughout menopause. While estrogen and progesterone levels fall, other hormones like follicle-stimulating hormone (FSH) and luteinizing hormone (LH) may rise. These hormonal variations can have an effect on numerous systems in the body, resulting in physical and psychological changes.

- Managing hormonal balance during menopause frequently necessitates a mix of lifestyle changes, hormone replacement therapy (HRT), and other medical interventions. Regular exercise, a balanced diet high in calcium and vitamin D, and stress management skills are examples of lifestyle improvements. For some women, HRT, which includes replacing hormones that the body no longer generates in sufficient amounts, can be successful in reducing symptoms. However, there are hazards, and pursuing HRT should be done in cooperation with a healthcare specialist.

- It's crucial to understand that menopause affects each woman differently, and the severity and duration of symptoms might vary. Furthermore, genetics, overall health, and lifestyle choices can all have an impact on the menopausal experience. Regular check-ups with a healthcare provider, open discussion about symptoms, and a personalized approach to management can assist women in navigating the hormonal changes associated with menopause and maintaining general well-being throughout this time of life.

Men's Hormonal Wellness

Men's hormonal health is an important component of overall health and vigor. Hormones influence a wide range of physiological activities, influencing anything from mood and energy levels to reproductive health.

Men must maintain hormonal balance in order to live a healthy and meaningful life.

Testosterone, the principal male sex hormone, is crucial to men's hormonal health. It has an impact on muscle mass, bone density, fat distribution, and the formation of red blood cells. Hormonal variations, on the other hand, can occur for a variety of causes, including aging, stress, bad lifestyle choices, and underlying health issues.

Elements and strategies for promoting men's hormonal wellness:

Physical activity has been demonstrated to increase testosterone levels and enhance hormonal balance. Aerobic and strength training both contribute to general well-being and can improve hormonal health.

A well-balanced diet is essential for hormone regulation. A diet high in important nutrients, such as vitamins and minerals, aids in hormone production and function. Adequate zinc, vitamin D, and omega-3 fatty acid intake is very critical for testosterone levels.

Adequate Sleep:

Adequate sleep is necessary for hormonal equilibrium. Sleep deprivation can disturb the body's natural hormonal rhythms, resulting in imbalances and potential health problems. Each night, aim for 7-9 hours of quality sleep.

Stress Management:

Chronic stress can raise cortisol levels, lowering testosterone production. Stress management practices such as meditation, deep breathing exercises, and hobbies can help reduce the impact of stress on hormonal health.

Keeping a Healthy Weight:

Obesity is linked to hormonal imbalances, namely a drop in testosterone levels. Adopting a healthy lifestyle that includes a balanced diet and frequent exercise can aid with weight maintenance and hormonal wellness.

Limiting Alcohol and Avoiding Excessive Smoking:

Excessive alcohol and smoking consumption might have a harmful impact on hormonal health. These habits, when moderated or eliminated, can contribute to overall well-being, including hormonal balance.

Regular medical check-ups are vital for monitoring hormonal levels and recognizing any potential problems early on. Consultation with a healthcare expert is essential for correct diagnosis and appropriate intervention if there are concerns about hormone abnormalities.

Relationship Health:
 Emotional well-being is inextricably linked to hormonal health. Strong, healthy connections and effective communication can help to reduce stress and maintain emotional equilibrium.

Strategies for Maintaining Hormonal Health in Men

A well-balanced diet:
Consume a well-balanced diet that is high in whole foods such as fruits, vegetables, lean proteins, and whole grains.
Make sure you get enough zinc, vitamin D, omega-3 fatty acids, and antioxidants because these are necessary for hormonal balance.

Exercise on a regular basis:

Participate in frequent physical activity, including both aerobic and strength training. Exercise aids in the regulation of insulin levels, the generation of testosterone, and the management of stress.

A good night's sleep:

Maintain a consistent sleep schedule and create a sleep-friendly atmosphere to prioritize quality sleep. Sleep deprivation can impair hormonal balance, particularly cortisol and growth hormone levels.

Stress Reduction:

To keep cortisol levels in line, try stress-reduction activities like meditation, deep breathing exercises, yoga, or mindfulness.

Chronic stress can have a severe impact on hormonal health, resulting in imbalances.

Keep a Healthy Weight:

Obesity and excess body fat can cause hormonal abnormalities, including low testosterone levels.

A healthy weight can be achieved through a combination of nutrition and frequent exercise.

Limit Endocrine Disruptor Exposure:

Keep an eye out for environmental elements that may contain endocrine disrupting chemicals, such as some plastics, pesticides, and chemicals in personal care items. When feasible, choose organic and natural goods to decrease your exposure to potentially dangerous ingredients.

Moderate Alcohol Intake:

Excessive alcohol use might disrupt hormonal balance. Limit your alcohol usage and be aware of its negative impacts on your overall health.

Smoking should be avoided:

Tobacco use has been linked to hormonal abnormalities, such as lower testosterone levels. Quitting smoking can improve your hormonal health.

Regular Health Examinations:

Schedule regular appointments with healthcare specialists to evaluate hormone levels and handle any abnormalities as soon as possible.

Consult a healthcare physician about any signs of hormone imbalance, such as exhaustion, changes in libido, or mood swings.

Useful Supplements:

If there are nutrient deficits, consider taking supplements. However, before beginning any supplementation, you should consult with a healthcare practitioner

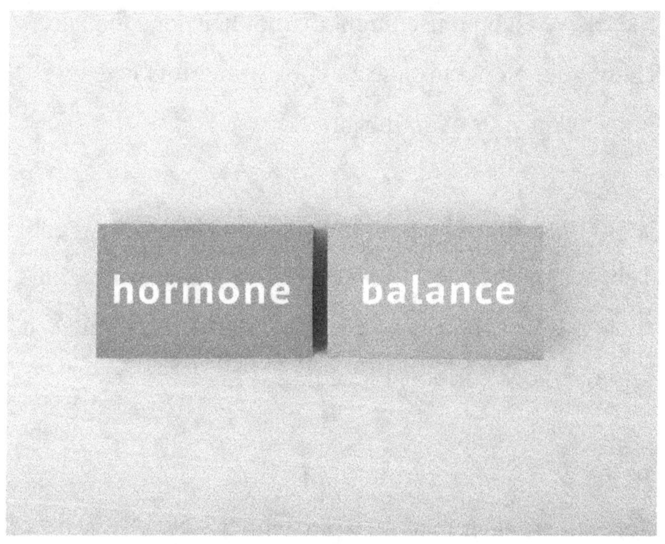

CHAPTER 7:
CONCLUSION

Resources and Further Reading

Alternative therapies, instructional materials, and supportive groups are among the modalities covered by these resources.

Access to resources that provide in-depth nutritional recommendations can be helpful in resolving hormone abnormalities. Books, online courses, and credible websites provide information on hormone-supportive diets, specific foods to include, and healthy lifestyle choices. Exploring publications written by nutritionists or medical specialists who specialize in hormone balancing can provide important insights into the function of nutrition in hormonal well-being.

Herbal Supplements: For decades, herbal supplements have been utilized to assist numerous areas of health, including hormone balance. Herbal medicine resources such as books, articles, and internet platforms can provide knowledge on plants known for their adaptogenic and hormone-regulating effects. However, before adopting herbal supplements into one's routine, it is critical to contact with a healthcare expert because they may interfere with drugs or have contraindications.

Mind-Body Practices: Stress management is critical for hormonal balance, and mind-body practices provide helpful stress-reduction methods. Meditation applications, yoga sessions, and mindfulness guides can all help people develop routines that enhance relaxation and mental well-being. These resources frequently include ways for controlling cortisol levels, a stress hormone.

Enrolling in educational classes or seminars focusing on hormonal health can provide individuals with understanding about the endocrine system and how it operates. Courses presented by professionals in the field on topics such as hormone imbalances, their causes, and evidence-based therapies may be available through online platforms, wellness centers, and educational institutions.

Investigating the knowledge of functional medicine practitioners can provide a personalized and holistic approach to hormone balancing. These healthcare specialists frequently investigate the underlying reasons of hormonal abnormalities, taking into account aspects such as nutrition, lifestyle, and environmental effects. Individuals can identify qualified specialists via resources such as functional medicine practitioner directories or recommendations from healthcare networks.

Joining online forums, support groups, or social media communities centered on hormonal health can foster a feeling of community and shared experiences. Individuals can use these channels to exchange information, seek guidance, and find encouragement. Engaging with individuals who have been through similar experiences can provide emotional support as well as practical knowledge.

Biofeedback and Wearable Technology: Individuals can monitor physiological markers related to hormone balance by using biofeedback devices and wearable technology. Resources that provide information on the most recent technologies, their accuracy, and their applicability in hormone tracking can empower people to take an active role in their health management.

www.ingramcontent.com/pod-product-compliance
Lightning Source LLC
Chambersburg PA
CBHW070848260726
48661CB00004B/1308